LEGACY

The NOW not anonymous diaries of a sperm donor

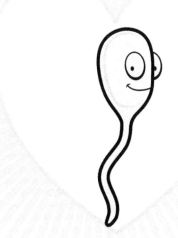

Kelly Clifford

KELLY CLIFFORD

Legacy

First published in 2020 by:

Profit in Focus Ltd
Registered Office: 82 Apollo Building, 1 Newton Place, London, E14 3TS
hello@profitinfocus.com
www.profitinfocus.com

Please note that this is the limited company through which I conduct my business, which has had no bearing on my motive for this writing this book. Any profits will be used to fund the Legacy6000 campaign.

Printed and bound by Ingram Spark/Lightning Source in the UK and in the USA.
Copy editing completed by Susan Andrewes – www.susanandrewes.com
Cover and interior design by Jon Wright Media - www.jonwrightmedia.com

ISBN 978-1-64633-835-1

The right of Kelly Clifford to be identified as the author of this work has been asserted in accordance with sections 77 and 78 of the Copyright, Design and Patents Act 1988.

A CIP catalogue record for this book is available from the British Library.

All rights reserved. No part of this book may be reproduced in any material form (including photocopying or storing in any medium by electronic means and whether or not transiently or incidentally to some other use of this publication) without the written permission of the copyright holder except in accordance with the provisions of the Copyright, Design and Patents Act 1988. Applications for the copyright holder's written permission to reproduce any part of this publication should be addressed to the publishers.

Copyright 2019 Kelly Clifford

Dedication

For my biological children.

KELLY CLIFFORD

Important Disclaimer

The contents of this diary are the personal thoughts and views of an individual embarking on the journey of becoming a sperm donor in the United Kingdom, and in no way constitute advice; nor will the contents necessarily always be precisely accurate.

If you are considering becoming a sperm donor, it is important that you research the rules and requirements of the country in which you live, as they vary significantly from country to country.

The area of sperm donation is complex and has far-reaching implications for the future. Make sure you seek out the right help and consider and explore all of these issues for yourself so that you can go into the process with your eyes wide open and having made a fully-informed decision.

Why I've written this book

What follows is the other side of the story. We often see things from the recipients' perspective, but often no thought is given to the thoughts and emotions experienced by donors.

I don't know whether the emotional journey I've been on is the norm or not. The reality is that it is not openly talked about. I know I had no one to talk to about my experience - someone who had already trodden this path - when I embarked on this journey. That needs to change, in my view, and this is my way of starting that conversation. Donors are not unemotional robots: we have emotions and feelings. My hope is that what I share gives you a taste of this in the journey that I have been on as a donor.

Most importantly, I share this for my biological children, so that in the event that something happens to me and we never get to meet, they know the story of how they came to be and how I felt about them.

The book is structured into four volumes. The first three are the original diaries that I wrote and published anonymously as a Kindle book on Amazon back in 2012/2013. They are still on Amazon today. The fourth volume is what happened next.

I know that there are differing views on the whole area of IVF, and I've no doubt that the decisions I've made may shock some people, divide opinion and inspire in equal measures. What I know for sure is that I can't live my life for other people. I can't be worried about their reactions. I can only live my truth, and this book is my truth - of which I am immensely proud.

KELLY CLIFFORD

Contents

Volume 1 - Inception	10
Volume 2 - Donation	28
Volume 3 - Dilemma	44
Volume 4 - What happened next	60

KELLY CLIFFORD

9 - Inception

Anonymous Diary of a Sperm Donor

Volume 1 - Inception

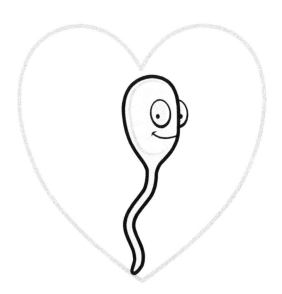

KELLY CLIFFORD

11 - Inception

Introduction

I think it is important that I be completely upfront about my reasons for writing this diary. Partly, it is to help me work through the complex issues associated with the path I have chosen to explore in becoming a sperm donor. Partly, it is to help raise awareness of the issue so that, if this diary helps some other man through the process or others to understand the journey, then it will have achieved its aim. Finally, it is to help document the journey so that I can share it with any biological children that result and tell them exactly how I was feeling each step of the way - should they choose to reach out to me when they turn 18.

As you will soon read in my diary, I have promised in my personal message to any children that result, that, should they wish to reach out to me, I will not deny them access to me; nor will I deny them the opportunity to understand more about their biological heritage. That is the promise I have made to both them and their parents.

I am an ordinary man looking to do what I consider to be an extraordinary thing in helping to create families that wouldn't otherwise be able to exist, by giving them the gift of a child. I am not so naïve as to think that the associated issues and opinions are simple or always supportive. I also know that the path ahead will not always be smooth.

What matters is that it is a journey upon which I am prepared to embark, despite any adverse views to which I know I will be subjected along the way.

I have deliberately kept identifying information vague and have not mentioned dates so as to preserve the anonymity of the process for the donor recipient and any children that may or may not result.

KELLY CLIFFORD

The lead-up

I'm a gay man and have long wrestled with the thought of having children. What I have now come to recognise is that there is very big difference between the romantic notion of having children and the actual reality of doing so. Many of my family and friends are having children and, despite the obvious joy that they experience, it has been almost unanimous that it is much harder than they ever expected it to be. I will say more about this later.

My partner of 10 years definitely doesn't want kids but for me it has never been a cut-and-dry discussion. Now, not everyone will agree with my views on the various issues, but that's okay. We are all entitled to our opinion. What is important is that I have decided on the best course of action for myself, when all factors have been taken into account.

Kids can be cruel

From my own experience, and I'm sure that of most, growing up isn't always easy and other kids can be cruel, especially when you don't fit in and don't conform. I know it is slightly different, but I experienced this growing up by being a fat child. I was teased and tormented, as you would expect. I also saw it time and time again with others who were considered to be different. Whether their family was richer or poorer, or depending on the clothes they wore or how they looked - basically anything that the kids could find to pick on, they would.

It could well be argued that that is a part of growing up, and I would agree with that, as my childhood experiences have definitely shaped the person I am today. I threw myself into my studies, at which I excelled, and am so grateful today that I did. Facebook and social media have really taken our lives by storm over the past few years and it is easier than it ever has been to re-connect with people we lost touch with years ago. What I find to be most interesting is that the kids who focussed on being 'cool' or on being part of the 'popular' crowd haven't achieved as much success as those kids who were considered different and who were tormented because of it. It's funny how life works.

Soul-searching for answers

It has taken a lot of soul-searching, but what I have realised is that it is unfair/almost selfish of me to bring a child into the world when they are different from the outset. How will they explain why they have two daddies, when everyone else seems to have a mummy and a daddy? Alright, I know that families come in all shapes and sizes in the modern age and that there is almost no such thing as a traditional nuclear family anymore. I also know that many will disagree with my view and argue that it is about loving and nurturing the child that matters most, but for me the traditional nuclear family ideal remains.

I grew up with two parents. I never experienced the impact of divorce. Our family is not perfect and I don't have the best relationship with my father, but I do have respect for the fact that they did the best job they could with what they knew at the time. Mistakes were made which have been forgiven but never forgotten. What it took me until my early twenties to realise was that my parents - and any parents for that matter - did the best they could with what they knew. No parenting manual is provided when a baby is born. Just as my Mum and Dad had to find their way, all parents have to do the same by trying different things to see what works and what doesn't. Making mistakes comes with the territory of being a parent and a tremendous amount of patience also.

Exploring the options

Going through this period of contemplation leading up to the decision to become a sperm donor, I explored many of the options available to us as a gay couple, including surrogacy, co-parenting and being a known donor. Many of these I didn't investigate after I really thought about the potential impact on the child, the practicalities, the longer-term implications if arrangements faltered and the difficult conversations that would be needed over time. None of these options sat right with me, but I wasn't able to articulate why until recently, when I stopped looking outwards for answers and started looking inwards. It's when I started looking inwards and got to the core of the issue that it became clearer.

One Sunday afternoon

Listening to Gaydar radio on a Sunday afternoon, doing some work on my laptop, an advert came on which talked about the possibility of becoming a sperm donor - helping to create families for people that were suffering from fertility problems as a result of cancer, accidents or otherwise. Hearing this instinctively made my ears prick up and stop what I was doing on my laptop.

I went to the website address they were advertising, had a read about what was involved and soon after completed the interest form. I figured that there was no harm in exploring what it entailed. The next day I received a response with a request to fill in a pre-assessment questionnaire.

Pre-assessment questionnaire

I scanned through the documents and, although there was nothing contentious, there was one thing that nearly stopped me from completing the form. It was something very small. It asked for the medical history of my mother and father. Although I was able to answer the medical questions, as I knew our family history, what I couldn't answer was my Mum and Dad's current weight and height. They were two simple, innocent words but it would mean that I would need to get the information from them to complete the form.

Remember that, at this point, nobody knew what I was contemplating doing. Not even my partner knew that I was exploring the potential suitability of my becoming a sperm donor. Of course, we had talked about it briefly in the past, but I wanted to know whether I 'passed muster' or not before raising the subject again.

So on one of my usual emails to my mother I slipped in that I was currently looking at setting up a critical illness insurance policy (I already have that in place for my partner and myself) and that I needed a few details from them. Mum sent through the information I needed without raising any suspicions, and so I had what I needed to complete the form and return it to the clinic for their preliminary consideration.

I didn't have to wait long for the answer: that same afternoon an email arrived saying that they would like me to come in for an appointment to digest all the information and decide whether or not I wanted to be a donor. At this appointment, a test semen analysis (including a test freeze/thaw) would be done.

The process

I would need to produce a semen sample at the unit so that the clinic could test how my sperm reacted to being frozen. For best results, I was told to abstain from sex or masturbation for at least two days, but no more than five days prior to my appointment.

It was explained that, shortly after my appointment, they would contact me to let me know whether or not I would be suitable to be a donor on the basis of my semen test freeze/thaw.

It was explained to me that the survival rate of sperm (approx. 50%) during the freeze/thaw procedure meant that not many men who volunteered as sperm donors were recruited, and to be aware that rejection as a sperm donor did not mean that I would be unable to have children naturally. Fewer than 1 in 15 men made it through the screening process to be a sperm donor.

Many potential sperm donors were rejected even though they already had children themselves. I was told that, if my semen analysis result potentially indicated a major problem, they would inform me of this, unless I specified otherwise.

If my initial test results were suitable, I would be asked to complete the legal consent forms required to be a donor and I would be required to attend a second appointment with one of their clinical team members.

At this appointment, the clinician would check through my forms and discuss any queries I may have. A quick physical examination would take place. Blood and urine samples would be taken, as a certain number of tests must be carried out to clear me of sexually-transmitted infections, including HIV, and to make sure that I did not carry any genetic abnormality.

I would be contacted with the results when they were available. It would take approximately 14 days for the results to be ready. Assuming all was okay, I would then be asked to attend a series of appointments to provide samples for storage.

The number of visits required would vary, but the average was 10 (over a two- to three-month period). After completing my donations I would again need to attend the clinic for the final physical examination and repeat the blood/urine screening. This would enable the clinic to complete the testing and quarantine requirements and to release the sperm for treatment.

It was strongly recommended that I consider counselling, as the issues involved were highly complex and far-reaching. It was explained that counselling was an opportunity to consider whether or not I wanted to proceed and to ask questions and clarify for myself what donation would actually mean for me.

The light bulb moment

We agreed on a mutually-convenient appointment time for the next week, some nine days later. I met with a close female friend the day after all this happened. As I had decided not to share what I was considering doing with my partner or any members of my family, it was a relief to talk to someone candidly about it without fear of being judged. My friend is also a coach, so she was very good at asking some very probing questions. It was just what I needed because it made everything click for me and slot into place.

What my friend helped me realise was that it was quite brave to be honest with yourself and admit that you didn't want to raise a child. Not everyone was cut out to be a parent and, being a first-time parent of a now 1-year-old child, she knew first-hand what it was like. It was far harder than she had ever envisaged and she was quite candid in admitting that there were times she wished she could be free again. Don't misunderstand, she dearly loves her child and has always wanted children, but I appreciated the realness of her admission.

You see, I have never had a yearning to have a child or to be a father; I am not really that drawn to babies or young children. Looking back on what I know my brother and I were like as children at times made me realise that it is the romantic notion of being a parent that keeps teasing me. What I now realise with clarity is that I have neither the will, the desire nor the patience required to raise a child. The reality is that I don't want to raise a child. I don't think it is in my DNA, so to speak, for many reasons. Some people have the demeanour and patience to be parents; I don't think I do.

You know what, I now realise that that is completely okay, and having this realisation is a huge relief. I don't want to raise a child, but many people do, but can't for many reasons. Being a parent is a largely very selfless act and if I have the missing link that could help these very people who dearly want to be parents achieve their dream of having a family, then that will fill me with immense joy and give extra meaning to my life.

The appointment

So after this really timely and insightful conversation with my friend, for which I will forever be grateful, I returned to my office and decided to move the appointment forward by six days. I needed to find out whether I was eligible or not. I couldn't bear waiting another week with the same thoughts and fears circling around my mind.

I don't know whether I am alone in thinking this, but I always had this secret fear that I was infertile. I don't know why, and it was completely irrational as there was no evidence to suggest it. If I'm honest, what worried me most about the appointment was discovering that I was infertile like the people I was trying to help and that the genetic testing would uncover something really nasty that had been lying undetected.

So I arrived at the clinic and registered at reception. The person with whom I was scheduled to meet was running 25 minutes behind schedule so sitting there in anticipation of what would unfold wasn't helping my nerves. After a few awkward jokes to break the ice, I soon felt at ease and was able to ask and have answered some of the questions I had around the legal implications, the process and, importantly for me, the typical profile of clients that would likely be using my sperm. I won't go in to details for anonymity purposes but I was reassured by the response. I was also reassured by the fact that I could elect to be notified when a child was born as a result. I wouldn't have any additional information than this but decided that I would like to know. I'm sure that this will raise a whole host of emotions when it happens but I will deal with this if and when it happens.

We spent a good 20 minutes just chatting. I was offered further counselling on numerous occasions throughout the consultation but declined, as I was okay with the progress so far. It then came time to produce the sample.

I was given a relatively large pot with a lid. I joked that if they expected me to fill it then they would be sorely disappointed. It was huge! This was a common misconception around volume about which I was instantly reassured. The whole experience was very clinical though. Let's just say that it wasn't an environment conducive to being 'inspired' if you were feeling too nervous. Thankfully, that has never been a problem for me. No stage fright for me: I have a good imagination!

Usually I would have left to await the results and the next appointment, but decided that, as I had already travelled for an hour to be at the clinic, I would hang around for another hour to get the results and then have the required blood and urine tests if successful.

I had produced my sample, screwed on the top of the pot and placed it in the chamber as instructed to do. I could do no more: the die had been cast, and I would have an hour to wait to find out whether I was fertile enough or, worst case, infertile.

Whilst slightly nervous, I decided that, whatever the outcome, as long as I had taken it as far as I could then that would be enough. If I didn't get through the screening then that would be okay; at least I would know that I had done everything I could.

The results

While I was waiting for the results I was able to speak with my consultant further and learn more about the process and the incredible work that the clinic does in helping to create families. Their approach is different to most other fertility clinics and they have an excellent success rate as a result.

I was open in sharing my secret fear about being infertile. My consultant recalled a time when he was studying at university: they were required to produce their own sample and look at it under the microscope. He said that, without exception, every male student had held their breath as they had looked into the microscope and that a collective sigh of relief had been audible when they had seen movement. This was reassuring - I was not alone in this irrational thinking. I almost felt as if it was the ultimate test of one's manhood. Crazy, I know. I commented that I felt like I was waiting for exam results. The consultant joked that he would be sure to bring them to me in an envelope, which made me smile.

The swing doors opened and in walked the consultant. "Do you want to come into the office and we'll go through them?", he asked. "Let's do it then", I responded. I was getting no sense either way from him as to whether they were good or bad.

He went through each of the factors they were looking for, as well as the baseline level required. I was above all of them, with one factor over four times the level required. I was secretly thrilled! What a relief: not only was I not infertile, I was potentially one of the less than 1 in 15 people suitable to be a sperm donor. The blood tests for genetic screening were the only remaining obstacle.

We completed the consent forms, which I had reviewed prior to the appointment to make sure that I was okay with everything. The only bits that I didn't complete related to a personal message to be given to the donor recipients and any child that may result. I wanted more time to think about this, as it was important to me that I take the time to leave a personal message of encouragement for the future. It would mean closure for me too. I'll say more on that later though.

The blood tests were taken and a urine test done. I can do no more. The 14-day wait for the results has begun. Fingers crossed that nothing negative from a genetic screening perspective is uncovered that has so far gone undiscovered. I feel like I am waiting for those damn exam results again!

A message with meaning

Earlier I mentioned that I had an opportunity to leave a message for both the donor recipients and any children that may result. This is important to me for many reasons. I wish I could share both messages with you verbatim but I fear that this would potentially compromise anonymity, so won't do so.

In short, I did impose a couple of conditions for the recipients that, if they weren't prepared to accept, then I would encourage them to do the right thing and look for an alternative donor. This is not something I can police so will have to rely on the integrity of the recipients. One condition was that they would be honest with the child as to how they came to be in the world. In my view, the child should be given the choice as to their reaction and not have it decided for them. The message I left for any potential children was what meant the most to me. I promised that I would not deny them access to me, if they wanted it, nor the opportunity to understand more about their biological heritage should they decide to reach out to me when they turn 18.

Why I want to be sperm donor

For me this is a purely selfless act: I want nothing in return. In fact, I have decided not even to receive the compensation offered for my clinic visits. It is not about the money whatsoever. I am doing this because I will potentially be able to give the ultimate gift to a couple who can't conceive naturally: the gift of a child!

Of course I am not so naïve as to think that it is easy as that. There are still many issues I have had to think about, including the decision not to tell my parents. I don't think they will understand, especially my Mum. She is a doting grandmother to my gorgeous 1-year-old niece. I think it would upset her immensely to know that there are children out there who are biologically her grandchildren but who she is not able to see grow up or even ever meet, unless they decide to get in touch with me when they are legally able to access my contact information in the UK at the age of 18 (or 16 if getting married).

I have even wrestled with whether or not I should tell my partner, as it will be at least 18 years before it impacts on us, should the child wish to get in touch. I have decided that I will chat to him after all of the test results have come back okay, giving me the green light to start the donation process. The decision will ultimately be mine, but I am expecting that my partner will be supportive, as this is something I really want to do.

It is a few days after the appointment and I have been doing some research on the internet. As you would expect, opinion is divided. Fertility rates are decreasing and IVF and fertility treatment are gaining wider acceptance. I was at the gym this morning and one fact caused me to hesitate for a moment. As part of this process, I am permitting the creation of up to 10 families from my sperm. If each family has two children then that means I could potentially have 20 biological children. Wow…how will I explain that to Mum if they all contact me at the age of 18?! I say that tongue-in-cheek now, but it is quite a concept to get your head around and, if I'm honest, it caused me more than a moment or two of hesitation.

As I continued with my workout and thought through the ramifications, I came back to my reasons for doing this. It is to help other couples achieve their dream of having a family. Helping to create up to 10 families by giving them the gift of a child.

What other people think doesn't matter. When I filter out the noise, that is what it boils down to. What greater gift can I give than the gift of life? That will be my ultimate legacy.

Next hurdles

So here I sit, finishing up my first diary. It is still 10 days until I get the results of the blood tests and there are so many thoughts bouncing around my mind. I don't want to get too far ahead of myself, just in case the results identify a problem. Yes, I am slightly nervous, but I'm only human, so that is understandable.

The three biggest things I will be thinking about over the next 10 days are as follows:

1. To what extent to tell my partner, if at all?

2. Whether I should in the future confide in my brother so that someone in my family knows, should something happen to me? If so, what is the right time to do this?

3. The firm hope that nothing negative comes back from the test results. That is out of my hands now.

I will release another diary update once the results have been received and share what I have decided on the other two thinking points. Be sure to look out for it if you are interested in sharing this journey with me. There will likely be many ups and downs over the coming period.

Wish me luck!

LEGACY

KELLY CLIFFORD

LEGACY

Anonymous Diary of a Sperm Donor

Volume 2 - Donation

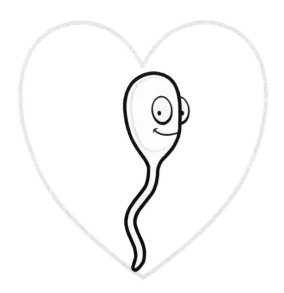

KELLY CLIFFORD

Picking up where I left off

In my first diary, Inception, I spoke of my decision to begin actively exploring the possibility of becoming a sperm donor, and shared with you both my thinking and the process I went through to see whether I would be eligible and meet the stringent health criteria required.

All initial test results from the clinic visit came back okay, and the test freeze/thaw of my sperm was successful. It was then time for the full blood screens to be done. I signed all of the consent forms. The wait for the results would be 10 days.

In my last diary I indicated that the three biggest things I would be thinking about over the next 10 days would be as follows:

1. To what extent to tell my partner, if at all?

2. Whether I should in the future confide in my brother so that someone in my family would know, should something happen to me? If so, what would be the right time to do this?

3. The firm hope that nothing negative would come back from the test results. That was now out of my hands.

The wait for results

As I write this part of the diary it is five days into the 10-day wait and I'm really surprised at how nervous I feel. I know from a health screening point of view that it would be unlikely for anything to come back abnormally, as I have been in a committed monogamous relationship for over 10 years. I don't know how it is for you, but the mind can play tricks on us. What is making this wait more difficult for me is the added layer of genetic and chromosomal testing involved.

I thought at the time that there would just be some routine blood tests but now the possibility has dawned on me that this genetic testing could uncover something seriously wrong with me, of which I am not currently aware. The results could change my life forever in an adverse way. I can't dwell on this though. It is out of my hands. What will be, will be.

Some decisions

On the partner front, I have decided that I will chat with him about it after the test results have come back and I know that I have passed all of the hurdles required to be a donor. I don't know why I feel nervous about doing this as it won't really have any impact upon us in the short or medium term; nor does it have to in the long term either. I think it is a case of having to fully come to terms with the reality of the situation myself in order to be confident and comfortable with my decision to do it.

The jury is still out as to whether to confide in my brother or not so that someone in the family knows. I certainly won't contemplate saying anything until a successful birth happens, but in any case I am getting ahead of myself by thinking like this, as it could all prove fruitless in five days time, depending on the test results.

The results are in

It is now five days on, all of the results are in and thankfully everything is okay. What a huge relief it is, as it has become more than just about being a sperm donor in my mind. I had no idea what would come back or be discovered and thankfully all is well. I am now cleared to start the donation process. Some of the results were back a few days ago but it was the genetic tests that took a bit longer.

The donation process

I now have to embark on the donation process, which typically involves 10 to 12 visits to the clinic. The target is to donate enough to fill approximately 60 straws. It follows that if the volume of each donation is larger than average, then fewer visits will be required. Sperm production volumes vary from man to man. We are all unique in every respect. We can't really control that bit!

There are restrictions that must be observed. For example, clinic visits should occur at least two days after the previous ejaculation but no longer than five days after the previous ejaculation. Alcohol has to be limited to no more than two units a day as it can damage the quality of sperm. I didn't expect it to be so prescriptive but I understand that it has to be that way so that the best quality sperm can be captured for use. This will take some planning and balancing as I have my own sex life to consider also!

Knowing this, I have made a decision which makes me laugh even as I write it: if I am going to be donating sperm then, DAMN IT, I am going donate the best quality sperm I can! I have today begun researching foods that enhance sperm production and improve quality. I want to produce SUPER SPERM!

Foods that are purported to help improve sperm count and volume

My internet research showed that a number of key vitamins and minerals are required to boost sperm production. With that in mind, I am undertaking to boost my intake of the main vitamins and minerals that are purported to help improve sperm count and volume.

Foods high in zinc

Zinc is essential to the healthy production of sperm. A deficiency in this trace mineral can lead to a low sperm count, poor motility and reduced production. Men with lowered sperm counts should thus make sure that their diet includes foods with an ample amount of zinc. These foods include beef, chicken, turkey, lamb, pork, crabmeat, lobster and salmon. Adequate amounts of zinc also can be gained from eating brown rice, pumpkin seeds, whole grain cereals, beans and peanuts.

My choices from this group are: chicken, turkey & whole-grain cereals.

Foods high in selenium

Selenium is an antioxidant that can improve the motility, shape and volume of sperm. Natural sources of selenium include Brazil nuts, walnuts, tuna, beef, chicken, eggs and cheese. However, one should take particular care when consuming selenium as too much of it can be toxic. According to some sources I have seen, an adult should eat no more than 400 micrograms of selenium a day.

My choices from this group are: chicken, tuna & eggs.

Foods high in vitamin C

Eating foods high in the antioxidant vitamin C can help improve sperm count and quality, as well as reduce a condition called 'agglutination', which is when sperm become clumped together. Foods high in vitamin C include such fruit as oranges, lemons, kiwi, papaya, mangoes and tomatoes. There are also plenty of vegetables high in vitamin C, such as broccoli and potatoes, and yellow, red and orange peppers.

My choices from this group are: broccoli, potatoes & tomatoes.

Foods high in L-arginine

L-arginine is one of the 20 amino acids that constitute protein and is essential to boosting sperm volume. It can be found in high-protein foods such as peanuts, Brazil nuts, pork, chicken, beef, turkey, seafood, soybeans and chickpeas.

My choices from this group are: chicken, turkey & seafood.

Foods high in vitamin E

Vitamin E is an antioxidant excellent at ridding the body of free radicals that can damage sperm. This vitamin has been understood to improve sperm volume and motility. Foods containing ample sources of vitamin E include wheat germ (particularly wheat germ oil), eggs, sweet potatoes, sunflower seeds, almonds, hazelnuts and peanuts.

My choices from this group are: wheat germ, eggs & sweet potatoes.

Foods high in folate

Numerous studies, including one reported in the Dutch journal "Fertility and Sterility", show that folate (folic acid) is vital in improving sperm concentration and quality. To increase your folate intake, eat plenty of leafy green vegetables, such as spinach and kale, as well as broccoli, lentils, chickpeas, organ meats, oysters, asparagus, oatmeal and avocados.

KELLY CLIFFORD

My choices from this group are: broccoli, asparagus & oatmeal.

I don't know whether anything will actually work or not to improve my sperm quality and volume, but I'm up for giving it a go. At least I will know that I did absolutely everything I could to ensure the best possible output. Now that the results are back, next on my list is to chat to my partner about what I want to do. How do you slip something like that into the conversation? Hmmm...!

Partner chat

In my previous diary, I spoke of how my partner of 10 years definitely doesn't want kids, but that for me it has never been cut and dry. We had spoken about this previously and at the time I had mentioned the possibility of becoming a sperm donor for a couple that couldn't otherwise have a family.

That conversation took place a couple of years ago but then life got in the way and I never really explored it any further. I have seen a close friend benefit from receiving donor eggs and donor sperm to create three beautiful children who are so wanted and completely loved. I guess it was when she decided to have her third child from stored embryos and I saw her around the time that she was going for IVF treatment that I started thinking about it again.

It was hearing the advert on the radio that re-ignited my interest further, and provided the final catalyst for action. For me it is about creating families that wouldn't otherwise exist. Just because I don't feel that I want to or can raise children for the reasons identified in my first diary, I don't want to deprive other couples of the chance to have a family that they so desperately want. I know that any children will be very loved.

The conversation with my partner was over in a flash and I honestly don't know why I was so worried. I think it was more to do with me than him. To be completely honest with you, there is a lot of head trash that comes with making a decision to do this. Things you don't expect. Since I have elected to be informed at each successful birth, I truly won't know how I will feel until that happens. Who can know? It's certainly not something most people ever experience - knowing that a child is biologically yours, but that you are not likely to see them until they are 18, and only if they choose to seek you out. To counter this, I have promised myself always to remember why I am doing this. I am confident that that will be my anchor through the ups and downs that I would be naïve to think won't happen.

My partner is completely supportive of my decision and is happy for me to do what makes me happy but obviously had some concerns around the legal and, particularly, the emotional implications. He just wants me to be absolutely sure of all the implications. It did cause me to stop and revisit my reasons and motives for wanting to do this. I did ask some further questions of the clinic to cover some of the legal questions I had on future liability, etc. I was happy with their responses, so have gone ahead and booked an appointment for my first donation clinic visit at the end of the week. There is no time like the present!

The first donation

Well, it is the day of the first donation and I was actually feeling really nervous this morning before my appointment at 8:00. It was probably a lot to do with the unknowns of the process itself.

The journey to the clinic from my home is 75 minutes each way by train, so it really will be a commitment if I have to make approx. 12 round trips over the ensuing weeks and/or months, which is what I am told is the average number of visits required. The train journey to the clinic was relatively trouble-free and I arrived at the clinic 10 minutes earlier than my 8am appointment. I elected for an early morning slot to get it out of the way and not run into scheduling delays at the clinic - we all know what it is like with scheduled doctors' appointments! I also wanted to ensure the least amount of disruption to my daily schedule.

So there I sat and sat....and sat some more. I waited for another 30 minutes beyond the appointment time, which was not helping with the nerves. I don't really know why I felt nervous. Perhaps it was the unknown. Sure, I had visited initially for testing but somehow I had thought that this would be different to that experience. In some ways, though, it was different, as I had passed all of the testing hurdles that had consumed my thinking at the time and dealt with the possibility that the genetic testing results would uncover something seriously wrong with me that had so far gone undetected.

I think mainly I was nervous because it had dawned on me that I was 'actually doing it'. The donation samples I was about to start giving over the ensuing weeks and possibly even months would be frozen and used in 'real' women to make 'real' babies and create 'real' families that otherwise wouldn't exist. These would be children I might never get to meet or know. All of these thoughts were running through my head and, whilst I remain certain of my decision to go down this route, I am human and do have emotions; so, on reflection, this morning I was bound to feel some anxiety and nervousness.

The clinician finally came in, called my name and led me to the laboratory where, after providing my name and birth date for identity checks and signing the consent form, I was duly handed one of - as I described in the first diary - the most inconveniently-designed screw top containers possible for the purpose. I guess for the clinic it is a trade-off between keeping costs down and serving the purpose for which it is intended. With my screw top container (with sharper edges) in hand, I proceeded to the 'donation' room.

Talk about an uninspiring environment. The 'reading' material was directed towards the straight male market and is something that would need to be addressed if the clinic were to attract more gay males, as they had set out to do with the campaign that prompted me to contact them in the first place. Luckily, not having 'material' was not an issue for me as my imagination was enough and soon I was done. I put the screw lid on the container and duly put the donation pot in the chamber between the corridor and the sterile lab. That was it, and off I went to the train station to catch the train back to London.

Timetabling donations

I felt what I would describe as really 'floaty' on my journey back to London. What I had chosen to embark on was beginning to really sink in and, in all honesty, I could understand if others would choose to opt out at this point - something they are well within their rights to do. The thought of another eleven early-morning starts and a three-hour return journey for just 10 minutes in the clinic (if they are on time) during the colder winter months made me wonder whether it was worth the hassle and inconvenience.

Twelve visits would mean a massive 36 hours of my time. It would also impact upon my life by having to limit alcohol, watch what I eat and manage when to have sex with my partner to fit in with the requirement for donations to be at least two days after a previous ejaculation but no more than five.

My thoughts kept looping back to why I am doing this, and the reasons far outweighed the inconvenience and sacrifice. I would urge any other man looking to do something similar to what I am doing to be very clear on WHY you are doing it: you will need it to refer back to as you go through the drudgery of donation over the ensuing weeks and possibly months.

When I got back to my office, I got my calendar out and looked at my schedule to work out how I could do this, aiming for two visits a week for balance. My plan for the donation period would assume sex with my partner on a Saturday night, and clinic visits on a Tuesday and Friday. It might sound calculated, but I think you have to be to get through this process with the least amount of disruption to your everyday life. It is not just me I need to consider but also the impact on my partner. As a result, I have scheduled the next six clinic visits and will reassess when I know how many more visits will be required.

It's late so I will finish writing now and head to bed. I will write again in a couple of weeks' time and update you on how the donations are progressing. Sweet dreams.

Some interesting sperm facts

Men are sperm-producing machines, knocking out an army of the little things every second. Here are the Top 10 Facts on sperm that I found when researching the internet:

1. An average man produces 1500 sperm per second and per testicle.

2. A sperm waggles its tail 800 times for every cm it moves forward.

3. 40-600 million sperm are released every ejaculation, depending on how long it was since the previous one.

4. The taste of semen is affected by what a man eats: fruit and sugary foods will make it taste sweeter, while red meat and dairy products will make it taste bitter.

5. A teaspoon of semen contains only 5-25 calories so is not very fattening if you swallow it.

6. Women who swallow sperm before getting pregnant are less at risk of complications during pregnancy. This is because the woman's immune system will recognise the sperm cells, decreasing the chance that her body will fight the foreign bodies that have just fertilised her egg.

7. Oysters and celery in particular have been said to help increase sperm production.

8. The average speed of an ejaculation is 31mph.

9. The average male ejaculates 7-10 inches.

10. Sperm can live on a toilet seat for up to three hours and inside a woman for up to five days.

A fortnight later

I have just returned from my fifth donation visit and early signs indicate that this could be the last visit. I went in with this expectation as the first visit yielded 11 straws for freezing, the second 12 straws (I'm particularly proud of that one) and the third 10 straws. These were all above the initial sample of nine straws so, who knows, my super sperm food diet might be working!

KELLY CLIFFORD

The target is for the clinic to have between 50 and 60 straws. I found out today, however, that I let myself down on the fourth visit, with only six straws. It's weird how you are quickly able to judge the size of your 'load': it did seem light when I did it. I remember thinking, "Is that it?" Hee hee. I had had a particularly stressful couple of days so I think there actually must be a direct link between stress and fertility and virility levels, if my experience is anything to go by.

It appears that one more visit will be needed to 'finish off the job', as today's visit yielded 10 straws, bringing us up to a total count of 49 straws after five visits. Thank goodness I won't have to make the originally-envisaged 12 visits as the journey is seriously wearing thin now. It is freezing in the mornings and if it wasn't for my firm reasons for doing this, I would probably have thrown in the towel by now, if I am completely honest about it.

I'm almost there and feel really proud of what I am doing to help create families that wouldn't necessarily otherwise exist. I feel proud for staying the course. Hopefully my last clinic visit will be on Tuesday, so I will write another diary and let you know how the final appointment goes, which I think will entail blood tests also. Happy weekend!

LEGACY

KELLY CLIFFORD

43 - Dilemma

LEGACY

Anonymous Diary of a Sperm Donor

Volume 3 - Dilemma

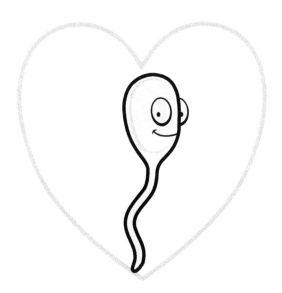

KELLY CLIFFORD

45 - Dilemma

Final donation

My last diary left off at the point where I had just completed my fifth donation visit to the clinic and thankfully was told that I had just one visit to go. Well, that day has arrived and I am just back from my visit.

Waking up this morning, it was a real relief just knowing that I wouldn't have to make this journey to the clinic ever again. Rather selfishly, the relief at not having to make the three-hour round trip for a 10 minute clinic visit twice a week outweighed the fact that I was edging nearer to having my sperm available for donor use.

The clinic visit started off as all the other visits had. It feels like déjà vu every time I make a visit because I end up sitting in the same chair in the waiting room, looking at the same surroundings, hearing the same radio station and waiting for the clinicians, who are always running late even at my appointment time of 8am. I still don't understand how a clinic can run late at the start of the day as consistently as this one has. This time, at least, I had to have a blood test after providing my final donation, which was something a little bit different to previous visits - just to mix things up a bit!

As far as I understand, once the results are back from this round of blood tests, in about one week's time, the samples will be in 'quarantine' for one full month, before being made available to potential recipients.

Reflecting back

The difference travelling back this time was that I felt relieved that the clinic visits are over but a bit overwhelmed, if I am honest, at the fact that it has become more and more real. Before long, there will be no turning back: up to this point I have been able to stop the process at any time. It is true that I can withdraw my consent at any time in the future, but that wouldn't apply to embryos already in vitro.

Reflecting on the last few weeks, it really is a surreal thought that in the storage freezer are about 60 straws of my sperm and that soon my characteristics will be listed for recipients to select or not. Although they will never get to see a picture of me, to help them decide, I wrote both the recipients and any children that result a letter, something I mentioned back in my first diary. I stand by what I wrote in imposing a couple of conditions on the recipients, conditions that, if they weren't prepared to accept, then I would encourage them to do the right thing and look for an alternative donor.

I still know that this is not something I can police, so will have to rely on the integrity of the recipients. One condition was around being honest with the child as to how they came to be in the world. In my view, the child should be given the choice as to their reaction and not have it decided for them. The message I left for any potential children was what meant the most to me. I promised that I would not deny them access to me, if they wanted it, nor the opportunity to understand more about their biological heritage should they decide to reach out to me at the age of 18. I will absolutely always stand by that commitment.

Test results

The test results came back a couple of days ago, and all is well. We are now in the one-month 'quarantine' period, after which the samples will be made available to potential recipients.

Over the past couple of days I have been really reflecting on this whole process and am starting to doubt a few decisions I have made. I think the fact that it has all become so real now has caused me to really look inwards and consider the emotional impact of some of my decisions on me, my family and any children that may result from this process.

I will do some further research into my concerns and will write again once I have collected my thoughts.

A dilemma

When I had my original appointment with the fertility clinic and signed the consent forms, I indicated that I would allow the maximum limit of 10 families to be created using my sperm, which could result in 20 or more children. That's a lot of children! I guess I didn't give it much thought because I was more focussed on the act of being a sperm donor than on the consequences of the result, if you know what I mean.

As I have now passed the final screening and donation hurdles and am nearing the end of my role in the process, it has really prompted me to think about my motives and the longer-term consequences of the decisions I am making now. There are references to various studies on the internet on the longer-term impact on sperm donor-conceived children and I read them with interest. I must say that I didn't think that some of the issues raised were big ones but there was one in particular that stood out for me. How would a child feel to be told that they are donor-conceived, only to find out that they have 20 other half-brothers or -sisters? Not very special, I suspect, and this would undoubtedly have a massive psychological impact on the child.

I have tried to address many of the longer-term impacts detailed in some of these studies by leaving a message for recipients, requesting that they be honest with any children about their origins, as well as for the children, promising among other things to welcome them with open arms when they are old enough. I would really love to share that message with you in this diary but I need to protect the families and the children who receive it. I am also not receiving any payment for the actual donations, which eliminates one of the areas in the reports about donor children struggling with the fact that money changed hands.

Respecting my family heritage

The other big issue I am grappling with is the impact of 20 or more biological children on my family tree. Can you picture it? A normal looking family tree with between two and four children per person, and then it gets to me and there are 20 children with different women - and that is only if I find out about them when the child reaches the appropriate age.

I need to be responsible, and whilst, in an ideal world, I would love to be able to help create as many families as possible, the reality and practicalities of the situation dictate that I need to think about it very carefully and maintain respect for the integrity of my family heritage as best I can. I will have to give further thought to this balance.

It is becoming clearer to me that 10 families is just too many, but I don't know whether to simply dismiss my thinking and just keep the consents the same or whether to alter them. Perhaps I am over-thinking it, but my mind keeps coming back to these issues. They bother me so they must be important and can't simply be ignored. I still have a bit of time left to decide.

Another blood test required

Arrgghh! I just received an email saying that I would need to visit the clinic again for a 'final' blood test as the month-long 'quarantine' period is up. I thought I was done! This will be the third round of blood tests.

LEGACY

Do I have any blood left to give?

I've booked the appointment for tomorrow morning to get it over and done with and out of the way. Over the past couple of weeks, the dilemma I spoke of earlier has been circling around my head and, having confided in someone else about it, who it turns out was adopted (something I hadn't known), I am much clearer on what I am going to do. I think I will mention it at the clinic visit tomorrow.

Final blood test

It was quite interesting today at my appointment. I didn't see the person I normally see as this visit was purely for a blood test. My dilemma was fresh in my mind. The nurse said that she thought it was a truly wonderful thing that I am doing, which I thought was really lovely of her to say. We started chatting and I opened up about my concerns; that although I was in no way changing my mind about being a donor, I was questioning the number of families I wanted to help create.

The clinic nurse was completely understanding of my dilemma. I think she agreed with me and offered to have my usual contact get in touch to discuss it. It felt really good to get it off my chest. My advice to anyone going through this process is to not try to deal with it all by yourself. This is a very personal journey but you do need to confide in someone to deal with the emotional and practical issues that I know come up. The act of donating is the easy part. It is the emotional element that took me completely by surprise.

I am now back in Central London, sitting in a Starbucks enjoying a coffee, having just sent the following email to the clinic requesting an amendment to my consents. My decision has been made as to the best way forward as I see it, balancing out all of the factors that are

KELLY CLIFFORD

important to me.

My email to the clinic;

Hi XXXXXXX,

Well, I am just back from giving the final blood samples so hopefully all will be well with them!

I have been thinking a lot about the way forward, now that we have hopefully come to the end of this process.

Whilst in an ideal world I would want to help create as many families as possible, I need to <u>act responsibly</u> by considering:

1. The impact on my hereditary family tree

2. The psychological welfare of the children if they were to find out they had 20 or 30 siblings. That's not fair on them at all and I feel that it could cause lasting damage!

3. The practicalities of being willing to meet them should they want to when they reach the appropriate age, as I have undertaken to do.

As such, I wish to formally amend my instructions to the following, with which I am comfortable:

"Creation of a maximum of three families, with an undertaking to allow at least two children for each family. Anything beyond this will need to be discussed as appropriate, to gain relevant permission or not".

This will mean that between three and six children should result.

Please confirm that my record has been updated to reflect my revised consent.

Best regards, Kelly

An email back from the clinic

Eleven days passed the final blood test and having sent the email, and I still hadn't had any confirmation back from the clinic, which I thought was odd given their previous responsiveness, so followed up with them. Apparently the original email was caught by SPAM filters! What a time for that to happen!

The email I received gave reassurance that my wishes and consents would always be upheld, but that they wanted to arrange a call to discuss some implications and clarifications of my decision. My heart sank a bit, thinking, 'What could they be?'

The phone call took place the next day and the implications centred on multiple births. It would be difficult to cap an absolute number at, say, two if triplets were born. Of course this was hypothetical, and they also said that, because of the approach the clinic takes, multiple births weren't common for their clients, although it was still possible.

So on the revised consent forms, I settled for simplicity, with a maximum of three families. I also did so on the basis that I would be notified with each successful birth, and that I would easily be able to change my consent at the appropriate time depending on what unfolded, etc. My personal undertaking still remains to allow at least two children per family, as I want the children to have a biological brother or sister to grow up with.

I have also received confirmation today that the final tests have come back fine and the samples are <u>NOW AVAILABLE FOR PATIENTS</u>. Eeeek!

KELLY CLIFFORD

Reflecting back over the past months

As I reflect back on the past couple of months and the emotional and physical process I have gone through, I realise that I have had three full rounds of blood tests, including genetic testing, which could have unearthed anything. Thankfully, nothing adverse was uncovered. I have now made a total of eight visits. I have made sacrifices in my everyday life so that I could, in my mind, produce the 'best sperm possible' for storage. I figure that's the least I could do on my part. After all, I want 'super babies' to result!

That's a total of 24 hours spent travelling to and from the clinic. For context, that is broadly comparable to a flight to Australia!

I have received no financial gain for doing this. It all is driven by my underlying wish to be a sperm donor. I am an ordinary man looking to do what I consider to be an extraordinary thing: to help create families that wouldn't otherwise exist, by giving them the gift of a child.

My top 10 tips

If you have read my diaries and are considering doing this yourself, or if you know someone that is considering exploring this as an option, here are my top 10 tips based on my experience over the past couple months.

1. **Be completely honest with yourself**

    If you can't be honest with yourself, who can you be honest with? Dig deep and explore how this decision will impact every area of your life - both now and in the future. Allow yourself to run different scenarios through your head and consider your reaction.

Remember, it is okay to recognise that this process isn't for you. It certainly won't be for everyone.

2. **Consider future implications**

    It is really important to consider the impact on your family and its heritage and, most importantly, the psychological impact on children born out of this process. I initially consented to the creation of the maximum of 10 families, which could have resulted in 20 or more children. Further in, I realised that this would decimate my family tree and be disrespectful to my ancestors. When this was combined with the possible psychological impact of any children learning that they had 20 or more half-brothers and - sisters, it made my decision to alter my consent to a maximum of three families a complete no-brainer. Also, if you have committed to embracing any children that reach out to you at the age of 18 when they can obtain your details, as I have, then you will need to consider the likely consequences of choosing this path as well.

3. **Consider the impact on your lifestyle**

    You need to consider the impact on your life, not only as you are going through the donation process but in the future too. The donation process became quite tedious for me as it entailed a three-hour return train journey for each visit to happen. You will need to make sacrifices through the donation process, which will have an impact on both you and your partner if you have one.

4. **Be prepared for unexpected emotions**

    We are human beings at the end of the day and, as such, emotional creatures. Going through a process like this will stir emotions that you would not ordinarily have to face. Be prepared for this, and make sure you explore what comes up head on. Don't ignore any element. It won't do you any good in the longer term.

5. **Find the right clinic**

   Not all fertility clinics have the same approach, so it is important to find a clinic that you feel comfortable with. I did not feel comfortable donating to a clinic that was involved in really invasive practices such as injecting a needle that contained the sperm into an egg. The clinic I chose advocates natural fertility as much as possible. They work with the cycle of the recipient and whilst the egg is fertilised in a petri dish, the sperm is not forced into the egg in an invasive way. They still have to break through the wall of the egg. The strongest swimmer still has to take the glory!

6. **Confide in someone that won't judge you**

   I started out this process keeping it all to myself and found it became easier when I confided in one or two others who I knew wouldn't judge what I was undertaking to do. They were a terrific sounding board as I was grappling with the issues that came up along the way for me. They all happen to think that I am doing a remarkable thing and I know they will continue to be there for me along the way.

   I have made the decision not to tell my Mum, as I wouldn't expect her to understand and I couldn't do that to her. I couldn't tell her that she has biological grandchildren whom she may never see, and certainly not until they are adults. That would be cruel, given that she dotes on my brother's daughter who is just over a year old as I write this. I might still tell my brother a bit further down the line just in case something happens to me. I want someone from my family to know that these children exist and might one day want to understand more about their biological heritage.

7. **Take the time to write a message for any children that might result**

    I think this is really important. In my message, I explained how this came about, why I am helping in this way, my dreams for their future, the sort of people I would want them to become and, importantly, an undertaking to not deny them access to me should they want it when they reach the right age. This has benefited me as much as I hope it will the child. I am not some uncaring monster that did this for money. I did this out of love and I wanted them and the recipients to know that. Put yourself in the child's position and treat them as you would want to be treated in their position.

8. **Be committed to see it through**

    Sacrifices will have to be made through the donation process, so be prepared for them. You must also be prepared to stay committed to seeing the process through. At times the easy option would have been to opt out. If you don't think you can stay the course, then don't start. It will save both time and expense for all parties involved.

9. **Discuss your concerns as the process ensues**

    Don't bottle anything up. If you have any issues or concerns along the way then voice those concerns. This is definitely a case of it being better out than in!

10. Always remember why you are doing it

This is one of the biggest things, in my view. Be clear about why you are doing it and keep this at the forefront of your mind. The journey won't necessarily be smooth, emotionally or practically. This is what has got me through the past couple of months, and I know it will see me through the challenges that will inevitably crop up in the future.

The road ahead

I am not so naïve as to think that this is the end of the journey. The road ahead remains uncertain, as I can't possibly know how I will react emotionally when I receive word that a baby has been born. Who could know? That will be my next real challenge, as I currently see it.

All I know is that, as long as I keep my reasons for doing this at the forefront of my mind, I will be able to work through anything. I know also that the people I have confided in will be there to support me should I need them to.

I just love the thought that, in a year from now, up to three babies might have been born and three families created. Sure, I won't see them for a very long time, nor possibly ever see them at all, but that is the sacrifice I am prepared to make, such is the conviction I have for what I have chosen to do.

My next diary

So here I end this diary, having navigated all the hurdles and challenges

LEGACY

in reaching this point, and with my samples now AVAILABLE for couples to choose when creating the family for which they long. My work is done, so to speak. I hope these diaries show that sperm donors aren't necessarily heartless, emotionless, self-serving machines - as some paint them out to be. It is quite the contrary in my case and, I'm sure, in many others. My next diary release will likely be in at least 12 months' time and only if I have news to share about successful births and how I have dealt with news of that. Fingers crossed for a successful outcome!

Thank you for sharing this journey with me.

KELLY CLIFFORD

59 - What Happened Next

LEGACY

Now Not Anonymous Diary of a Sperm Donor

Volume 4 - What happened next

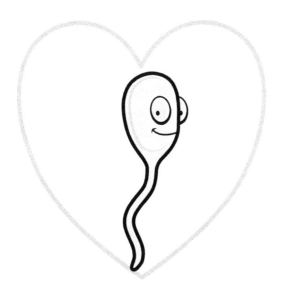

KELLY CLIFFORD

61 - What Happened Next

LEGACY

So, fast forward to today – over six years on!

It's really interesting looking back at my original diaries and at how I had hoped to have news within the year. That was completely unrealistic. I had just assumed that my samples would be used soon afterwards, and didn't expect what would actually happen.

In this volume, I am going to step back to that point and progressively write about the stages that followed, with all the emotional ups and downs they brought with them.

The wait begins

I decided early on that I would maintain an ACTIVE interest in the process and keep in regular touch with the clinic. The first year passed and I anxiously emailed the clinic asking if there were any pregnancies or births. After all, a pregnancy lasts nine months, so I thought that there would be a strong possibility of something happening.

When the news came back that not only were there no pregnancies, but that none of my samples had even been used, I was so disappointed, I wanted to understand why. Upon further enquiry, I was told that the clinic had just brought in a large batch of samples from Europe, so had a big supply of samples to work their way through. In some respects, I felt let down by this news; given the emotional journey I had been on to even get to the point of donation, and given my understanding that there had been a shortage and that they needed donors to meet demand, this felt really deflating.

There was nothing I could do though so, in the meantime, I simply got on with life, with it never far from my thoughts.

Questioning my choice of clinic

Another six months passed by and I emailed the clinic again (which I tend to do twice a year) for an update, only to learn that still none of my samples had been used. Disappointing news again.

At this point, I began to question whether I had chosen the right clinic. Would they ever use them? Should I withdraw my permission and donate again with another clinic? My head was swirling with these questions and more.

I ultimately decided at that point to give them another 12 months, concluding that, if nothing resulted, then I would go through the process again elsewhere. I was becoming more and more emotionally invested in the outcome.

The final chance

When I sent another email, I had low expectations but remained hopeful of some news. I had deliberately left the gap between follow-ups longer and had tried to put it out of my mind in the meantime. My focus turned in the interim to creating a business legacy by defining a BIG MISSION to help 100,000 small businesses globally grow their profits. To serve this scale of audience, this meant creating an online technology solution from scratch.

This is something I'm passionate about doing, as more profit means more choice for small business owners. In my eyes, this ultimately means they can do more 'good', whether that is by employing more people, by creating abundance for themselves and those around them or by giving back.

Unexpected news

As I said, I had low expectations and expected the same response as on previous occasions. The difference this time was that it was my final chance for the clinic to have at least used my samples for one patient. That would be enough for me to stay with the same clinic and not donate again elsewhere.

I remember the morning very well. I was to have a full day ahead on the tech build, which was nearing an important milestone, and it had been a week or so since I had sent the email requesting an update. An email appeared and it was from the clinic. It said the following:

```
2nd February 2016

Dear Kelly,

I can confirm we have 2 on-going pregnancies with your samples.

Best wishes

xxx
```

Mind officially blown

To receive the news of not just one, but two pregnancies completely blew my mind. Two families were in the process of being created. What a wonderful message to receive. Since they were early on in their pregnancies, I knew that there was still a long way to go and that anything could happen over the course of the pregnancy. I needed to keep my expectations grounded.

It doesn't stop your mind wandering though. I'm obviously not told any of the specifics of due dates etc., other than there is a LIVE pregnancy. I could only assume that they were both in the first trimester. Right then and over the coming months I found myself googling the size of the foetus at each stage, right from a jelly bean through to a watermelon.

In a weird way, this brought me a lot of comfort and enabled me to feel a part of the process that a complete stranger was going through with my biological child.

With a rough idea of the dates, I suspected that both would be born by the end of 2016 and that there was therefore no point in following up in the meantime. In hindsight, I wonder if I was afraid to follow up out of fear that both pregnancies had been lost. I wanted to stay in that little bubble of hope that everything would be okay for both families and that healthy bundles of joy would result for them.

An unexpected twist

I knew that, if everything had gone well, it would be within the window for birth, so I followed up a bit more frequently at that point. On 26th September 2016 the email arrived. There had been a LIVE birth. As this was the first time, I didn't know how much I would be told, and had to clarify. All I can be told legally is the year of birth, the sex and if all is well with mother and baby.

The news was in, and my first biological child was a little GIRL - but the twist was that she was born in 2015. Huh?! How was that possible? A year earlier than expected? How did that happen?

It transpires that I was misinformed about the stage of the first pregnancy. Looking back at the updates received etc., and working back,

I suspect she was born in December 2015, but have no way of knowing for certain.

There was absolutely no reason to be disappointed about being misinformed, as it was completely overshadowed by the absolute JOY and DELIGHT I felt. I had a biological daughter. WOW!!!

A deluge of emotions

This news was huge for me and the reality dawned again that I would not be able to know, see or share experiences with her for at least the next 18 years, and only then if she wanted to know me and reach out to me. How did this make me feel? Had I made a mistake? Had I underestimated the emotional burden of this news?

I wasn't sure at first, and spent the first few days working my way through the news. It was front and centre of my mind constantly. I gave myself space to really think about it. I re-read my diaries and revisited my reasons for doing it in the first place. And you know what? I was fine with it.

The biggest emotions I felt were pure LOVE and JOY. Love for this little part of me that I may never get to meet, but also pure JOY that she was now in the world and being nurtured and cared for by a family that dearly wanted her. My heart was singing This news came just as I was about to travel back for a holiday to Australia, following a five-year absence. I had thought about telling my brother on the trip but it was the first time that I would meet my nieces and it just didn't feel right for many reasons, so I decided against it at the last minute.

I was a little apprehensive meeting my nieces for the first time, and wondered in particular what emotions it would stir within me regarding my own choices. In the end, however, it wasn't an issue. Don't misunderstand, I LOVED meeting them but, if anything, it reinforced my view that raising children is just not for me.

Seeing my parents interact with their grandchildren, however, was very confronting and confusing. They loved and adored them. How would they react to this news that they had another grandchild confirmed and another one on the way, whom they might never get to meet?

It was a huge emotional burden to carry and, once the words had left my mouth, I wouldn't be able to un-tell them the news. There would be no putting that genie back in the bottle. In the end, I decided that I would wait, that there was no rush, and that I would at least wait until the second child was confirmed. My Mum was also due to visit me in the UK that following May, so I had time to think about it more. What I did know was that, if I did decide to share the news with my parents, then it would have to be FACE to FACE. Something like this was TOO BIG to be shared in any other way.

Tick tock, tick tock

There can often be a lag between a child being born and the clinic being notified of the birth by the parents. The desire to know that the child has arrived safely and that both mother and child are well has been really strong for me, given the suspicion that the child is due around a specific time window but not knowing the outcome until months later. My email frequency to the clinic increased substantially during this 'waiting' window to once every couple of weeks. I felt disappointed with every email that came back saying that there was still no news.

BLUE!

On 21st April 2017 an email arrived with the news that my second biological child to a different family had been born, and that it was a BOY. I had secretly hoped that it would be a boy, given that the first was a girl. One of each! Wow!

It's really funny how your mind can work sometimes. In some warped way, it felt like the family name could live on, as my brother has two girls whose name is likely to change when they get married (although it might not of course, should they choose), when the reality is that they would never have my family name.

What made this special in a different way for me (but no less than the first) was the thought of another me of the same sex growing up. I wondered if he looked like me. I wondered if he had my same blue eyes. I wondered if he had the same curly dark brown hair I had when I was young. I wondered if he would think like me and have other similar traits.

For both, I have become intrigued about the 'nurture' versus 'nature' debate. Which personality traits and behaviours are genetic and which are learned? This would be the ultimate test, should I one day have the fortunate opportunity to meet them.

Sharing the news

Given that I had decided at this point not to tell my family, thinking that my parents would not understand, it was really important that, should something happen to me or to my partner, they would have a way of knowing the truth - especially now with the arrival of my biological daughter and son.

KELLY CLIFFORD

I had no idea what I expected people's reactions to be on hearing the news but kept it to only a handful of people who didn't know each other, but who were in some way connected. This would mean that they would be able to make contact with my parents should something happen to me.

I spent hours thinking about what I would say and re-read the message over and over again until it got to the point where I just thought, "screw it, just do it" and sent the messages. What came back was so supportive, it made me really grateful to have these special people in my life. These people would be the guardians of my legacy, and that gave me real comfort.

```
Hi XXX,

You may not understand what I am about to share, but here goes….

For various reasons, we decided that we didn't want to raise
children in a two-father setting as we didn't think it was fair,
as childhood is tough enough without added adversity.

But I still had a strong pull to want to be a biological father
so I decided that I wanted to turn it into something positive
and set a personal mission to help create three families that
wouldn't otherwise exist without my help (helping people
suffering from infertility due to cancer treatment etc.).

So a few years ago I became an anonymous sperm donor (although
by law in the UK my identity would become known to them at the
age of 18 should they choose to reach out to me).

Well…the big secret is that I have two biological children that
I won't likely meet for at least 18 years to two different
families.

A little girl was born around Nov 2015 (I am only given the
birth year but have deduced the approximate month from various
```

LEGACY

emails) and today it was confirmed that a baby boy to a second family was born in Sept 2016 (around the time we were visiting Oz!). I knew about the little girl when I saw you but didn't have any confirmation on the second birth except I knew it was imminent. There is often a six-month lag time between birth and the records being updated on the registry.

There was actually a third pregnancy at the start of this year to a third family but sadly they miscarried. I have given permission for three families to be created - no more than that.

For obvious reasons, I didn't think it fair to tell Mum and Dad as I think it would be too tough for them (especially Mum) to know but not be able to see them etc.

So I have effectively 'outsourced' the child raising part :o) hee hee. Hopefully I will be lucky enough to meet them and become part of their lives when they turn 18. It gives me such a warm feeling of joy to know that I have helped create these families that wouldn't have otherwise existed and there are two little 'me's' out there, which secures my personal legacy.

If something ever happens to me then please make sure my parents know about this and I'll keep you updated on any more arrivals.

Big love

Kx

KELLY CLIFFORD

Telling Mum

Every couple of years, Mum comes across for a trip to the UK, when we get to spend two weeks of quality time together. Mum's next trip followed hot on the news of baby number two, so I didn't want to lose the opportunity to potentially tell her.

I thought long and hard about the best approach and what I decided was to break it down into two components, the first the fact that I am a sperm donor (without giving the outcome), and the second the outcome. As I mentioned earlier, this sort of news is not something you can un-tell someone, so I needed to make sure that it was Mum's choice to know or not.

The first part was to share the original three diaries (included at the start) with her, together with the letter I left with the clinic for the recipients and any children that may result. This would be step one in the process.

The day arrived when I decided to do it, as we were heading out for a day of sightseeing together, just the two of us. We started talking about how it is hard sometimes being on the other wide of the world and about how she sometimes feels that we aren't as connected as she would like. I apologised for that as I am completely rubbish at keeping in touch regularly, but also said that there was a reason for it, in that there was part of me that I hadn't shared. I told her that I didn't want there to be anything left unsaid between us, especially as we got older. Losing two family members over the course of that year had reinforced just how precious life was, so this was really important to me.

I reassured her that it was nothing to be concerned about, but said that I would message her some diaries which I wanted her to read and digest,

LEGACY

and that we would discuss it afterwards, when I would answer any questions she might have.

I knew that Mum would read them straight away, so waited nervously until she emerged from her room. Of course, I didn't know that she was definitely reading them, but I had a strong suspicion that she was!

Some time later, she emerged from the room, came up to me and gave me a big hug, telling me that she was proud of me. When we had spoken earlier, I had given her the choice to know more or not, and had encouraged her to take her time to decide because it wasn't something I could take back once I told her. She agreed to do that.

An understandable but disappointing response

The next day, Mum and I picked up the conversation. She had a number of questions, which I answered. The words then came: "I would prefer not to know the outcome", the reason being the emotional aspect, which I completely understand. She would never be able to interact with them the way she does with her two grandchildren by my brother and his wife.

Let me be clear, this in no way reflects negatively on my Mum, who has always been fully supportive. Rather, it was an emotional reaction to the news that she had just heard. I told her that, should there be anything that results, then I would be open with her about it, but that it had to be her choice whether to know or not first. In typical Mum style, which I'm sure is the case for other mums too, she tried to fish a bit more, but I wasn't biting and deliberately kept it neutral. The choice had to be made first.

We pretty much left it at that. I completely respect Mum's choice, but still felt disappointed. Surely, she would want to know? I would want to know. Perhaps in time that would change. That was my hope anyway. She would be visiting again in two years' time, so I made a mental note to pick up the conversation again then if she didn't want to know any sooner.

Starting a Christmas tradition

From the moment that I heard the news of my biological children, and as the sex of each had been confirmed, the following Christmas I bought four decorations (two of each) and began placing them on the Christmas tree as part of what I plan to make an annual thing.

In my mind, I have this lovely thought of one day meeting each of them and being able to give them one of the two in the set of the decorations as a token, to demonstrate that I have been with them every Christmas, if only in thought. That not a Christmas has passed where I haven't thought of them and wondered what they are doing with their families. Hoping that they are happy. Hoping that they are healthy. But always knowing that they are loved.

A miscarriage

About a year passed and, as part of my regular check-in with the clinic, the news came back that only in that last fortnight my sample had been used for a third family and they were pregnant, albeit in the very early stages. I was delighted with the news and said that I would follow up in a couple of months' time, just to check that they had got through the first trimester okay.

When the news came back that they had miscarried, it felt like a punch to the gut. I felt incredibly sad – both for the family and for myself. I didn't expect to feel like that. I felt the loss of this little soul, a life unlived, a little piece of me that would never get a chance to thrive. They wouldn't get a chance to make their dent in the world. I just hoped that the family would try again when they felt able to repair the hole that I knew would be in their heart, as it was in mine.

A summer surprise

A further six months passed and it was in the summer of 2018 when news came in that the third family had tried again, were pregnant and that all was well. I was completely elated. Could my mission of helping to create three families that wouldn't otherwise exist without my help really be about to come true?

```
Kelly

I am delighted to say a third person is now pregnant.

Regards, XXX
```

It was at this point that something in me changed. I no longer wanted to hide this secret that I had been carrying. I was finding myself avoiding idle chit chat with new people, when the conversation inevitably turned to the notorious question: "Do you have any kids?"

My old response was always to say "No", which tended to close the conversation down. Increasingly, however, this was feeling disingenuous and wrong. It felt like, that by denying it, I was in some way denying my biological children's existence. This just didn't feel right, and so, with that in mind, I started being open about it on a selective basis, as a way of testing the water.

An unexpected response

People do surprise sometimes and I can honestly say that I haven't had one adverse response: people genuinely feel that what I have chosen to do is a great gift to the families. They all know people and other couples that suffer from fertility issues, but this is something that people just don't tend to discuss openly.

The countdown begins

From what I could piece together from my email dates and from the responses, this third child would be due to be born in December 2018. All I could do now was wait and hope that the pregnancy progressed without any issues.

What was different this time was that I had a very strong instinct that this one would be a boy. I don't know why. I already have one of each, so the sex didn't matter so much to me. All I wanted was for mother and baby to be well. The feeling that it would be a boy never left over the ensuing months.

Christmas and New Year passed and, if everything had gone according to plan, then the new bundle of joy should have arrived. I mentioned previously that there is often a lag between a child being born and the clinic being notified by the parents of the birth. The lag in finding out is the bit that I have found most frustrating.

Once 2019 arrived, my email frequency to the clinic again increased substantially to once every couple of weeks. The feeling of disappointment with every email that came back saying that there was still no news remained.

8th March 2019

This day is one of the most memorable and proudest days of my life so far. It will forever be a very special day. Most people that know me will know that my partner and I became proud owners of our DREAM property in London on this date. It is a split-level penthouse on the Thames near Canary Wharf with panoramic views of the city. It's truly incredible and our 'forever' property in London.

It felt like the hard work, sacrifice and ups and downs over recent years in pursuing what we are each most passionate about professionally have been completely worth it, just for the feeling we had on that day. To say we were very happy is the hugest understatement.

But what almost no-one knew, apart from a handful of people, is that I also had a very special email arrive in my inbox that made the day even more special.

```
Dear Kelly,

We have now three confirmed live births. Congratulations!!

Best regards, XXX
```

```
Dear XXX,

I'm really keen to know the sex of the third birth, please. Are
mother and baby doing well and are they healthy, if you know
that too?

Thanks in advance for your further response. I'm thrilled with
the news!!!

Best regards, Kelly
```

KELLY CLIFFORD

Dear Kelly,

The third birth is male, born 2018. All good for the family.

Best regards, XXX

Thank you so much!!!

Absolutely delighted to hear that.

Best regards, Kelly

Wow... it had happened. And another boy, too! The legacy I had set out to create over six years ago was secured, and I had helped to create three families that wouldn't otherwise exist.

I have one biological daughter and two biological sons across three families! Being able to write this just puts the BIGGEST smile on my face. I know that feeling will never go away and I know that whatever happens next, these three precious little people are in this world because of the journey I went on and the decisions I made over six years ago to create a legacy and to help make difference for three families.

Seeing young families

I quite often find myself observing young families where the children are about the age my biological children are, and wonder what they are doing right now. This is never from a place of feeling that I am missing out, but out of curiosity for what they are like, what they are experiencing and how their individual personalities are developing.

Telling my family

I mentioned that, when my Mum last visited, I shared with her the first three diaries about being an anonymous sperm donor, but without giving any indication of the outcome. I also gave her the choice of knowing the outcome or not. She disappointingly, but understandably, said that, from an emotional perspective, she didn't want to know.

Fast forward two years and Mum was visiting the UK from Australia. It was the first time we had been together in the same location since then. To me, this is not something you talk about by email or Skype but something that needs to be done face-to-face. It's for this reason that I had chosen not to push it in the interim, but I had a growing sense in the lead-up to her visit that I would have to force the issue, and needed her to know.

For me, it felt like a whole part of my life was being kept a secret and that therefore I was not living 'my truth'. This is something I am very proud of and my family needs to know, whether they accept it or not. It is better that the truth is out than being effectively back in the closet - as I was before 'coming out' as gay to my family over 18 years ago. My thinking was that this couldn't be as big as having to deal with that, and therefore that, in time, they would come to accept it.

I refuse to live my life for others, and this is a core part of who I am and the legacy I want to leave. I felt that by keeping it a secret from them, I was not only denying the existence of my biological children, something which bothered me greatly, but that I was also living a lie.

It was for all of these reasons that, one way or other, Mum would know the truth by the end of her two-week stay.

KELLY CLIFFORD

Tensions building

Mum arrived for her visit and all was well. I decided to wait until the later part of her trip to broach the topic but hoped that she would raise it sooner. I didn't want to risk spoiling our quality time together, in the event that her reaction was adverse. When Mum didn't broach the topic, I found myself feeling a bit wound up and wondering why. Had she not thought about it? Did she not want to know? All sorts of unhelpful questions started circulating in my mind. This was not about Mum, but my reaction to it. I guess my nervousness about it all was playing itself out as doubt and frustration.

The day arrived

It was a Thursday and Mum would be flying out the next Sunday, so I decided that today was the day that I was going to raise it with her. My partner was out for the morning, so it was just the two of us. It was now or never. We were both sitting in the lounge and I knew it was time, so I asked the question, "Mum, have you had a chance to think about what we discussed last time - about being a sperm donor? Do you have any further thoughts about it?"

To my absolute astonishment, she replied immediately, "Yes, I have. I've thought about it a lot since then and I've decided that I want to know". There was no hesitation. Something like this can never be untold, so I asked if she was sure, and she said, "Yes, I am". I was completely taken aback, and all that was left to do was to say it and so I did. "I have a biological daughter and two biological sons across three different families." She broke out into a smile and seemed genuinely pleased with the news.

I reassured her that there would be no more families than the three families I had given permission for, but that there could be more kids should those families want to have further children. I haven't restricted that from happening as I believe it important that the donor families have the option of full siblings, should they choose.

We spoke about telling Dad and my brother, and agreed a plan. I'm not going to go into detail beyond this out of respect for them, other than to say that everyone now knows and is processing it in their own way. It certainly hasn't been an adverse reaction in any way, but time is needed for it to truly sink in. I need to give them time and space, and this is something that I am prepared to do. I am just feeling completely relieved that it is all out in open though.

A weight has been lifted

I didn't realise how heavily the secret had been weighing on my mind. Telling Mum, and having it be received well, created an instant release. I suddenly felt lighter in general about it all. The truth was out. There are no more secrets. It was now a whole new world of awareness and acceptance. This all put a big smile on my face.

I guess it is like anything: you don't realise the toll something has taken until the pressure is removed. I only wished I had done it sooner, but the reality is that I couldn't really have done so. I believe I've been respectful and given time where needed, but I am also relieved and thrilled that is now all out in the open.

I am not so naïve as to think that there won't be any future hurdles to get over, or any emotional fallout from my family, but right now it feels good. My biological children are no longer a secret to my family. That makes my heart sing.

KELLY CLIFFORD

To my biological children

As I mentioned at the beginning, my main reason for sharing these diaries was to tell the other side of the story. If, for any reason, my biological children and I don't get the opportunity to meet, then they will have the opportunity to know my story, where they come from and how I felt about them. As such, in this final section, I am going to speak to them directly in the form of a letter about my hopes and dreams for their futures.

Hi XXXX,

I have a picture of the future in my mind. It is of the day we get to meet. I know that it may or may not happen in reality but the thought gives me joy and makes me smile. I know that I won't be there to see you grow up and it is your Mum and Dad's role to love, nurture and care for you, but I hope a future exists where I can be involved in some way in your life.

I hope to be involved in your life in some way and to be able to watch your children, my biological grandchildren, grow up. I hope we get to make our own special memories together. I know that I will never be your Dad in your heart - that role is already taken - but here are ten things I want for you:

1. Don't hide your flaws

Share your dark secrets. Sometimes this may be difficult, but it's important not to bottle up negativity. You need to face your darkness, which we all have within us, so that it doesn't consume you. It's okay not to be okay. Don't be afraid to ask for help when you need it. You need to feel embarrassed at times in order to become more courageous and confident.

2. Do a little cherry-picking

Some people are going to disappoint you. It's important to

accept people as they are, but it's also important to choose the people with whom you surround yourself - it's okay to outgrow friends.

3. Enjoy being a child

Enjoy your childhood, even when there are times you wish you were a grown-up. Believe me, there are so many grown-ups who wish they had a second chance at childhood. This is a special time for new experiences, learning new things, learning to do things better and also to have fun and goof around. Don't forget the fun part. It is the stuff that wonderful memories are made of and will get you through any difficult time later in life.

4. Be in the moment and take long walks

Don't only love people when they are sick. Don't only forgive people once they've apologised. Enjoy life while it is happening - be present. You'll also learn a lot about yourself with a blank page or a quiet path. Learning to do things in solidarity will help you grow and open your soul.

5. Believe in something

Believe in something greater than yourself. I hope you find something to be a constant reminder of how lucky you are simply to be. I also hope you recognise and acknowledge that, whatever you believe, believing alone is not enough. You must fight laziness, open your eyes and work to find your own way.

6. Be good to yourself

Don't be afraid of being alone and don't be afraid of failure. Exercise regularly. Try not to smoke. Nothing is forever, so enjoy and appreciate. I hope you grow to be confident in your own skin and accepting of your imperfections, because they are what make you unique.

7. Love yourself

Happiness does not come from accomplishments, high moments or connections. It all goes back to the start… I hope you grow to fall in love with yourself wholeheartedly, to really appreciate all that you are and have been blessed with, to know that there will never be anyone else who can shine like you. I hope you never forget this. I hope you learn to be vulnerable and have an open heart in making real and meaningful connections but never risk your own happiness at the expense of another. Relationships matter.

8. Be kind to your parents

Your Mum and Dad will inevitably make mistakes. There is no manual that comes with raising a child. They are learning as they go. Cut them some slack. They are trying their best but will get it wrong sometimes. Know that their choices for you are coming from a place of love and of wanting what is best for you.

9. Accept that life is a roller-coaster

I hope you learn that this journey is going to get rough, but the highs overcompensate for those times; they are the moments I ask you to hold onto those close to you, because when the hard times come, these will be your light out of the tunnel.

10. Dream big

Imagination is your greatest gift. Never lose your imagination, even if others may poke fun at you. They can't see the miracles and magic unfolding in your head and they can't see the places to which your adventures take you. Never let anything stand in the way of your dreaming because you will lose focus. You will wake up filled with regret and excuses in your pocket. Don't let life pass you by.

Know that I will be there for you with open arms and an open heart should you want to meet me in future, no matter what. I

LEGACY

wonder what your passions are, what music you listen to or what your laugh will sound like. What I do know without meeting you yet is that there is no one quite like you — now or ever again. We are all unique. Embrace your uniqueness, whatever that is. You have everything inside of you that you need to go wherever you want to go and be whatever you want to be.

I will think of you every single day of my life as you grow into your own unique person. Don't change, be true to yourself and just evolve into all that you are destined to become.

Until the day we hopefully meet, know that I love you and that my heart sings at the thought of just knowing that you are in this world.

Your biological father,

Kelly

xxx

KELLY CLIFFORD

Launch of Legacy 6000!

With my personal legacy now secured, I want to make an even bigger impact so that my biological children can be truly proud of me. With the launch of this book, I am THRILLED to be launching my Legacy 6000 initiative. Without further ado, here's my new focus:

Mission

To inspire the creation of at least 6,000 families that wouldn't otherwise exist as a result of anonymous sperm and egg donation.

How

By raising awareness, inspiring people and providing a support community for at least 2,000 caring and selfless donors who have each permitted the creation of up to three families from their donations to create their own 'gift-of-a-family' legacy.

Your support

Help spread the word:

Website: Legacy6000.com
Twitter: @legacy6000_
Facebook Group: @legacy6000

Lightning Source UK Ltd.
Milton Keynes UK
UKHW020936220120
357413UK00011B/934